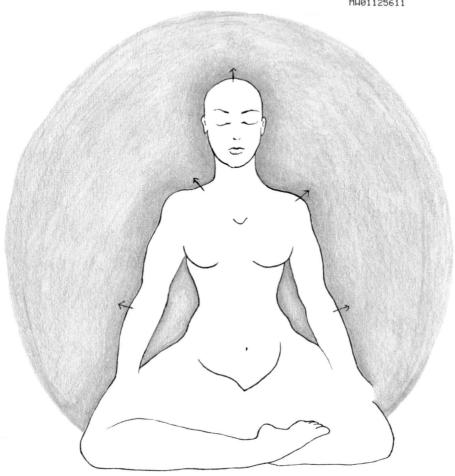

REIKI AS A SPIRITUAL PRACTICE
an illustrated guide

Nathalie Jaspar

Printed in the United States of America
First printing, 2018
ISBN-13: 978-1983423543

Dive Into Reiki
90 Hudson Street, #7B
New York, NY
www.DiveIntoReiki.com

*To Rebecca Spath
with love and gratitude.*

contents

foreword

Reiki as a Spiritual Practice: An Illustrated Guide is a wonderful book. First of all, Nathalie writes from her own personal, direct experience of having practiced these meditation practices. We can know something intellectually, but to really understand what the practices are about, we need to do them on a daily basis. Having worked with Nathalie over the years in my classes and retreats, I have seen how she has grown and developed a solid personal practice. This can be seen in her beautiful artwork. The drawings provide clear instructions on how to practice. There are many ways of teaching: we can teach in an auditory way, in a kinesthetic way and in a visual way. Nathalie's imagery is stunning, simple and to the point, which makes it easily understood by visual people like me.

I hope you will enjoy this book as much as I do and that it brings you a deeper understanding of the system of Reiki and how to practice.

Frans Stiene
Haarlem, Netherlands, July 9, 2018
Author of *The Inner Heart of Reiki: Rediscovering Your True Self* and *Reiki Insights*

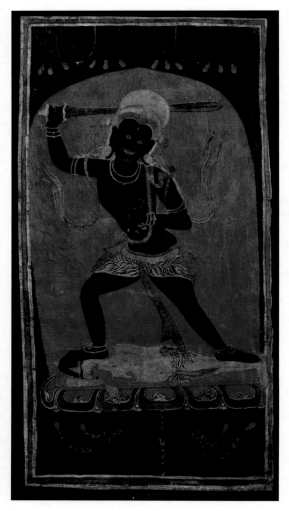

"Kyo dakewa
Ikaru na
Shinpai suna
Kansha shite
Gyo o hageme
Hito ni shinsetsu ni"

For today only:
Do not anger.
Do not worry.
Be grateful.
Practice diligently.
Be compassionate to yourself
and others.

Image: Arya Achala, Tibet, 12th century, Kadam Lineage, Collection of Shelley &
Donald Rubin. Rubin Museum of Art, Public Domain, via Wikimedia Commons.

the inspiration

It was the mid-2000s. I was browsing the Net to keep boredom at bay and, on a whim, typed "healing" in the search box. "Reiki practice" came up.

I had never heard of it.

The information available on Reiki at that time was based mostly on Hawayo Takata's version, Mrs. Takata being the woman who introduced this Japanese spiritual practice to the United States just after World War II. Reiki was explained as primarily a hands-on healing modality originating from a quasi-Christ-like enlightenment experienced by its founder, Mikao Usui, in the early 1900s.

There were also many outlandish theories, my favorite being that Jesus was an alien who brought Reiki practice to Earth—with not even a *soupçon* of a link to Japanese culture.

I was intrigued. And confused.

Given that I was cash-poor and totally ignorant of the practice, my first step to learning more was watching a YouTube video, in which the master gave a distant attunement (or connection) to Reiki energy overnight: I was to wake up with the ability to heal using my hands. I know, I know... But I thought it was just wonderful! I left my name in the video's comment section, as requested, and went to bed with a feeling of anticipation reminiscent of Christmas Eve when I was a child.

The next morning I woke up and nothing had changed. (You are allowed to say "Duh!") I felt the same as usual. No hot palms. No power to heal in seconds my frequent headaches. Nada.

My next step was to take a class. There were not many teachers around at that time. Eventually I found a woman who gave a one-morning course, was conveniently located and charged a reasonable fee. All factors that impressed me. The class lasted less than three hours. I received an attunement—performed in a rush without explanation—a copy of the Reiki precepts, a homemade-looking certificate and a lesson on the hands position to use when doing a Reiki treatment on another person. That was all.

In hindsight, I can see that the teacher had minimal experience—she was following her notes to give the attunement—and was nervous. She was thrilled when the class concluded, releasing me into the world thinking that, from then on, I could heal anything.

Which naturally didn't happen.

Weird things *did* happen, though.

My hands would become warm sometimes, especially in the subway. I could no longer tolerate crowds (I had never enjoyed them to begin with). And the idea that there was more to this "Reiki thing" kept crossing my mind.

I took another class, and this time the experience was unforgettable. The attunement gave me my first taste of interconnection with everything, and showed me how nurturing, warm and healing Reiki can be as a practice. Most of the class was once more about how to heal others. Reiki I and II were taught in one weekend, which meant that many of the teachings were rushed. But still, that doesn't explain why we were not shown a self-care protocol or even told that the basis of Reiki is self-care.

The first time I heard about the importance of daily Reiki practice on myself was when I attended the JCC Reiki Clinic with Reiki master Pamela Miles, who is down-to-earth, warm and nurturing. The clinics helped me get a sense of structure for my Reiki practice. There was and is—at time of writing, this Reiki clinic is still thriving—a sense of simplicity and respect that felt completely refreshing and which I had not found until then.

From that moment on I focused on taking lengthier classes, digging deeper into the self-care aspect of Reiki practice. I was lucky to complete my Level III training with Deborah Flanagan at the Center for True Health, in Manhattan. Flanagan trained in both traditional Japanese and Western Reiki and served as the perfect bridge for me to cross over to the traditional Japanese practice.

Through her, I discovered many techniques and meditations I continue to practice today. She also introduced me to Frans Stiene, a Reiki master who has studied the spiritual roots of the practice in Japan, and with whom I still study today.

I'm aware that the reason my road to finding the kind of teaching I needed was so long and winding was in large part my own doing: I approached the practice with a kind of superhero mentality, expecting to master it immediately. I was naive at best.

Reiki practice is, as the name indicates, a practice. One that must be approached with respect, discipline and an open heart and mind. One that has many tools, so that no matter what our personality or learning style is, we can find something that truly resonates with us and allows us to go deeper and deeper.

That's why this book illustrates only self-care techniques. They are the cornerstone of Reiki practice. When we heal ourselves, we are healing the world.

what you'll find in this book

Although I've included the basics of what Reiki practice is and a brief history of it, the book focuses on offering illustrated how-tos for common Reiki modalities of self-healing: meditations, breathing techniques, visualizations and, of course, the hands-on healing self-care protocol.

It has options for all levels of Reiki training.

What you won't find is guidance on how to share the practice with others (through sessions or attunements). And that is intentional.

I struggled to get a daily self-care routine going. A big part of the challenge was that I lacked the tools to implement a routine that could evolve with my practice. Some Reiki classes didn't include many techniques beyond hands-on healing. Other trainings offered plenty, but these teachings were hard for me to remember or to follow using written description. The more I chatted with other Reiki practitioners, the more I felt the need for simpler, more visual explanations of the most popular Reiki meditation techniques. So I started illustrating them. The result is this guide.

a caveat

My drawing style is rooted in my training as a painter at The Art Students League of New York. It's visual and graphic, and I don't incorporate clothing or hair in the human figures I draw. This doesn't mean you need to be naked (or shave your head) to practice Reiki or to receive a Reiki treatment. Reiki treatments and meditations are conducted fully clothed.

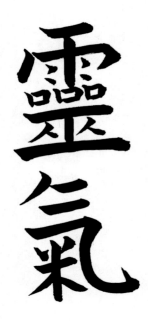

what's reiki?

The word "Reiki" is composed of two Japanese kanji:

Rei (meaning spiritual, sacred)
and
Ki (meaning energy, life force)

Together these kanjis mean "spiritual energy." Everything alive has Reiki. For me, this concept is equivalent to the theory in quantum physics that all the energy and matter that was released during the Big Bang created our universe. We all come from the same source.

The Reiki system is a nonreligious, spiritual one; its practice allows you to connect consciously with the ki, promoting balance, healing and well-being. It's a nurturing, relaxing practice that, over time, helps you let go of anger and worry and makes you feel interconnected, joyful and grounded in your everyday life.

The ultimate goal of Reiki practice is to rediscover your true essence (i.e., non-duality, coming from the same universal source).

what it's not

- A magical, super healing power.
- A quick fix.
- A guarantee nothing will ever go wrong.
- A manifestation tool.
- A practice focused only on the healing of others (rather, self-practice is the cornerstone of Reiki practice).

components

Although Reiki practice is known mostly as a hands-on healing modality, the traditional Japanese practice includes:

- Reiki precepts, or Gokai
- Meditations and techniques
- Four mantras and symbols
- Hands-on healing (on self and others)
- Attunement, or Reiju

benefits

Embodying your true essence may take a long time, but many benefits of practicing Reiki can be felt within a short time. Reiki—

- Relaxes and helps shift your nervous system from sympathetic mode (fight or flight) to parasympathetic mode (rest and digest).
- Accelerates the healing process and boosts the immune system.
- Improves wellness (e.g., better sleep, improved digestion, less pain).
- Makes you feel more balanced, grounded and centered.
- Reduces anxiety, anger and drama.
- Gives you more clarity, joy and confidence.
- Encourages a heightened feeling of connection, and a more meaningful life.

a brief history

The system of Reiki originated with Mikao Usui. Born in Japan in 1865, Usui was trained in esoteric Buddhism to the level of a lay monk.

Drawing on his spiritual experience, Usui created a system of teaching he believed would benefit anyone, religious or not. It would provide a method of interconnection in a time when the Industrial Revolution was creating a sense of alienation in Japanese society. His spiritual influences included Tendai Mikkyō Buddhism, Shinto- ism, martial arts and Shugendō. The basic premise was that healing exists within each person. The essence of the teachings, therefore, was self-practice.

The first teachings Usui gave to his students were the Gokai, or precepts. Then followed meditation and mantras. Usui was not known as a healer until later, when people felt healed from his teach- ings and from his practices, such as attunements (Reijus).

In around 1925, Usui formalized his teachings in order to make them accessible to even those inexperienced with energy work.

After his death, his former students formed a society, which they called Usui Reiki Ryôhô Gakkai. It spread to many cities in Japan, where members would meet to practice the techniques under the head teachers.

Chûjiro Hayashi, the teacher from whom most current West- ern lineages can be traced, studied in one of these centers, before opening his own in 1930.

From 1936 to 1938, an American-born Japanese woman named Hawayo Takata studied with him, later bringing the teachings to America. Takata learned from Hayashi a practical palm-healing technique, which is the basis of the current Reiki practice we in the West know today.

After Takata's death in 1980, her students established their own practices. Many of these students were influenced by the New Age trend, which is why most Reiki teachings now include the aura and chakra system—as opposed to the original Japanese practice, which uses only three energy centers.

Individual masters started to add their personal touches, and nowadays there are many interpretations of what Reiki practice is. Takata's student Barbara Weber Ray, for example, created the Ra- diance Technique, which has seven levels instead of the traditional three. Another student, William Lee Rand, created Karuna Reiki and Holy Fire Reiki, which are meant to attune the practitioner to higher levels of energy.

In truth, there is no best or strongest Reiki. There are only different people with different structural needs when following a practice.

What started as a Japanese spiritual practice is increasingly an accepted form of complementary healing in hospitals settings and private practices, from LA and New York to Buenos Aires, Madrid and Paris. It's also experiencing a revival in Japan.

levels of reiki training

Traditionally, Reiki training comprises three levels (although some Reiki teachers divide Shinpiden into two, for a total of four levels).

Reiki I (Shoden)
The beginning of the journey. Focuses on healing the self and on the basics of healing others.

Reiki II (Okuden)
Students learn three mantras and symbols that aid in focusing energy. They learn to work with Earth, Heaven and Heart ki, as well as learning the basics of developing a professional treatment practice.

Reiki III (Shinpiden)
Students learn the fourth mantra and symbol and how to perform attunements. They move deeper into their practice, exploring how they relate to themselves and to the universe. Eventually they may develop a professional teaching practice.

the precepts

The Reiki precepts, or Gokai, are one of the five elements of Reiki and can be considered the foundation of the whole system. They are guidelines for conduct and the first step in the student's process of self-healing.

It's believed that Mikao Usui introduced the precepts as early as 1915. The precepts in Japanese are—

Kyo dakewa
Ikaru na
Shinpai suna
Kansha shite
Gyo o hageme
Hito ni shinsetsu ni

Because Japanese kanjis can be interpreted in many ways, there are numerous versions of the precepts in English. Here are two of my favorite and most widely used translations:

version 1

Today only:
Do not anger.
Do not worry.
Be grateful.
Practice diligently.
Show compassion to yourself and others.

version 2

Do not bear anger, for anger is an illusion.
Do not be worried, fear is a distraction.
Be true to your way and your being.
Show compassion to yourself and others
because this is your essence.

Emulate the version that resonates most with you.

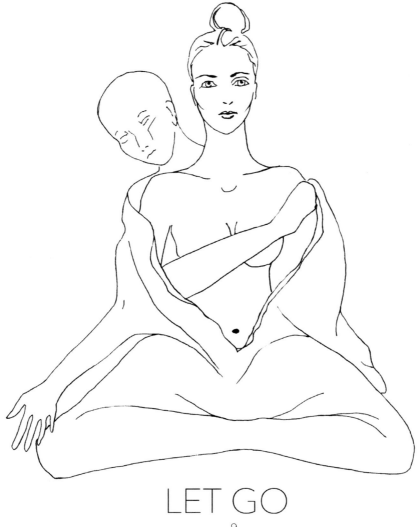

LET GO

embodying the precepts

I was on my way to a freelance writing gig. One I usually liked a lot, but not that day. Although I had been pretty good at hitting the right tone in the copy I wrote and the client was happy with it, in the last project I had failed miserably. As I exited the subway and walked toward the office, I felt extremely anxious. My heart was beating like crazy, and my brain was going at a thousand miles per hour. So I decided to sit down for a few minutes in a park—which was tiny, and situated between two giant buildings. I put on my headphones, closed my eyes and started meditating on the precepts—specifically, "Do not worry"—breathing deeply into my Hara.

After a couple of minutes, I could already feel the difference. My brain had slowed down. I could feel the fear moving through my entire body, but I felt it more from the perspective of an observer than anything. I kept breathing. And it came to me that fear was not allowing me to see beyond what I wanted. That I was defending myself instead of trying to understand the situation calmly. That I was taking feedback on my writing as an attack on my person. I began to breathe with much more ease. And suddenly I understood what was going wrong with the writing and how I could have a productive dialogue with my client from a more caring place. So I went to the office, sat calmly in the meeting room (despite the tension in the air) and explained what I believed was the misunderstanding and how we might approach it. We all relaxed, and after a couple of hours, we had the results we wanted.

It wasn't until that day, really, that I "got" at all levels the precepts as a meditation tool. I think that, in part, my Judeo-Christian background made me view them as commandments, which made me resistant to practicing with them. I would get angry at myself for being angry (because I was not supposed to feel angry). Or I'd feel guilty about being worried. It never occurred to me to use these feelings as guidance on how to integrate my Reiki practice into my everyday life.

how to work with the precepts

When you first start working with the precepts, it's best to focus on one line at a time (e.g., "Do not anger" or "Do not worry"). After a while, combine them and see how they relate to each other.

visualization

Place hands in Gassho (see page 14). Imagine a pond in front of you. The precept line is a stone you throw into the water, creating ripples. Notice what comes up for you.

using your body

Place hands in Gassho (see page 14). Choose one precept and repeat it silently. What do you feel or sense within yourself? Notice any change in your body. Is there a physical tightness or opening? Do you feel any old emotion coming up? Sit and observe. Do not judge or try to fix or manipulate what comes up. Just observe it and then let it go: stop repeating the precept and stay for a few breaths in the energetic space you created.

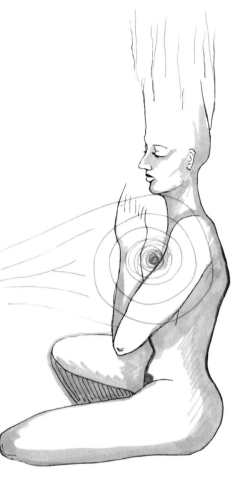

chanting

You can chant the precepts in Japanese as well, if you like. The vibration of the words will shake your thorax (where most of the body's organs are located), helping to release tension. When chanting, inhale all the way to the Hara and chant from there. (You may want to watch a video on YouTube of how it's done.) It requires a bit of practice to do properly, but it's an excellent way to settle a restless mind.

the 3 energy centers

Unlike Western Reiki practice, which often works with the concept of chakras, traditional Japanese Reiki practice focuses on three energy, or ki, centers:

Earth ki (Hara, 2 to 3 inches below the navel)
This energetic center represents the energy you were born with. It's your link to life and purpose. When this center is balanced and strong, you feel grounded and calm, and see things as they are.

Heaven ki (forehead)
The energetic center represents your connection with your spirit. It's related to inspiration, intuition and psychic abilities. When this center is balanced and strong, your vision is expanded.

Heart ki (heart area)
This energetic center represents your connection with others and with emotions. It is associated with learning and life processes. When your Earth ki and Heaven ki are balanced, your heart energetic center opens, and you feel your connection with every living being and with the universe.

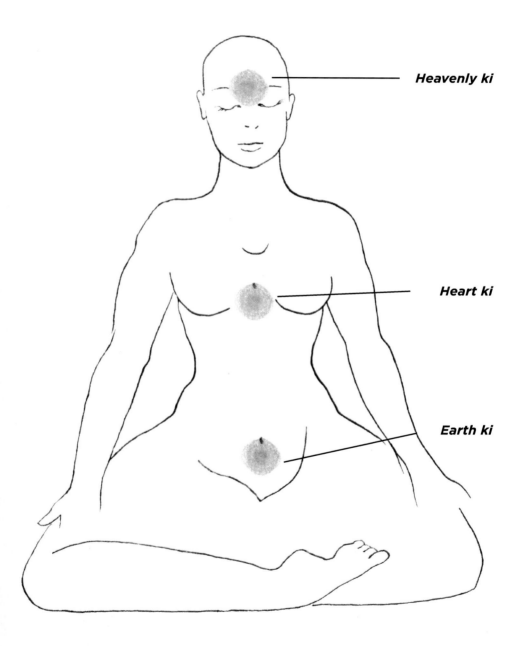

Heavenly ki

Heart ki

Earth ki

gassho

"Gassho" means "to place the two palms together." It's a concept similar to Namaste, but beyond honoring the true self that is in all of us, it also involves bringing our different sides together—left and right, female and male, darkness and light—and uniting the mind. It centers us and points us toward wholeness. When we feel whole, we heal. We stop acting from need and start acting from a more compassionate place.

how-to

1. Slightly press your palms together in front of your heart, fingers straight.

2. Keep the elbows from touching the body; the forearms are not quite parallel to the ground.

3. Keep one fist distance between the fingers and the tip of the nose.

4. Keep your eyes on the tips of your middle fingers.

You can use Gassho to:

1.   Meditate:
        a.   Recite the precepts.
        b.   Keep your eyes on your fingertips, inhaling while visualizing a white light entering your heart area through your fingertips, then exhaling the white light out.

2.   Center yourself and set your intent before practicing self-healing or meditation.

3.   End a self-healing treatment or meditation, stating your gratitude for everything you received during your practice.

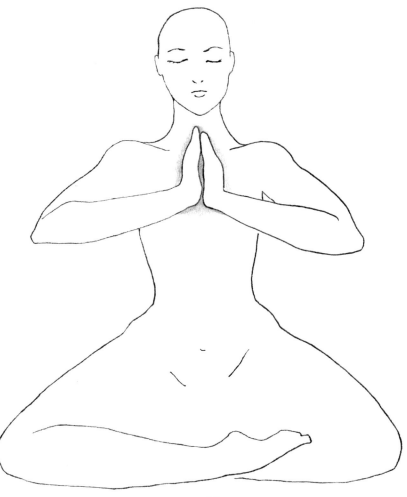

kenyoku hô (dry bathing)

Kenyoku Hô, or Dry Bathing, is based on Japanese purification rituals, traditionally done with water before entering temples. Although Western Reiki practice uses Dry Bathing as a modality of cleansing ourselves of negative vibes, in traditional Japanese Reiki practice, this purification modality focuses on cleansing negative thought patterns caused by fear, worry and anger.

It anchors you in your body and grounds you while activating several meridians (such as lung and heart). It's typically practiced before and after hands-on healing sessions (both on oneself and others, as well as before and after Reijus). I also use it before and after meditations.

There are many theories as to why we swipe twice from left to right, yet only once from right to left (see how-to, page 17), ranging from this giving extra energetic support to the liver, to it being based in the traditional cleansing techniques of monks before entering the temples, where they washed their left hand twice. There is no definitive answer.

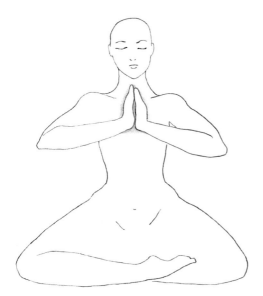

1. Place your hands in Gassho to set your intention to perform Kenyoku Hô.

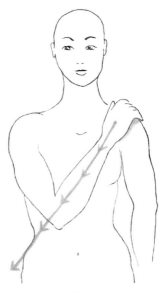

2a. Place your right hand on the left shoulder. Inhale and, on the exhale, sweep your right hand downward diagonally from the left shoulder to the right hip.

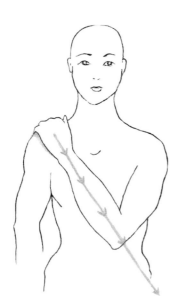

2b. Inhale and place your left hand on the right shoulder. Exhale and sweep your left hand downward diagonally from the right shoulder to the left hip.

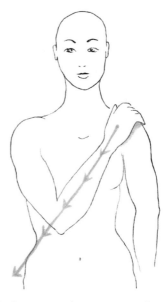

2c. Inhale, returning your right hand to the left shoulder. On the exhale, sweep your right hand downward diagonally from the left shoulder to the right hip.

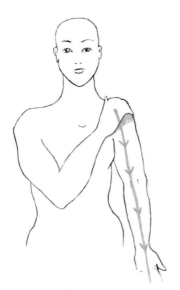

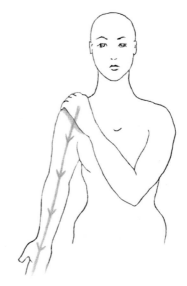

3a. With the left elbow against your side and your arm perpendicular to the ground, place your right hand on the left shoulder. Inhale and exhale, sweeping downward to the left fingertips.

3b. With the right elbow against your side and arm perpendicular to the ground, place your left hand on the right shoulder. Inhale and exhale, sweeping downward to the right fingertips.

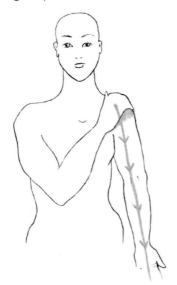

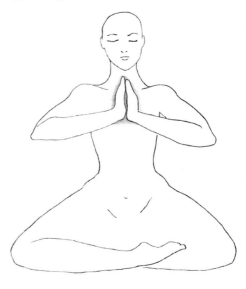

3c. With the left elbow against your side and your arm perpendicular to the ground, place your right hand on the left shoulder. Inhale and exhale, sweeping downward to the left fingertips.

4. Close with Gassho, to give thanks.

joshin kokyu hô

Joshin Kokyu Hô is used to focus the mind, clear the meridians and build energy in the Hara. In English, this practice is called Purifying Breath because, over time, it helps us to let go of anger and worry.

1.   Sit on a chair with your back straight and feet planted firmly on the ground, or cross-legged on the ground or in seiza (kneeling on the ground, your legs folded underneath your thighs while the buttocks rest on the heels). Place your hands in Gassho to set your intention to perform Joshin Kokyu Hô. (See page 20).

2.   Close your eyes and place your hands on your thighs, palms facing upward.

3.   Inhale and feel the energy coming in through the nose and moving down to the Hara.

4.   Pause, feeling the energy filling your entire body.

5.   Exhale, expanding the energy out of the body through every pore, into your surroundings.

6.   Repeat steps 3 to 5 as many times as you wish.

7.   Close with Gassho, to give thanks.

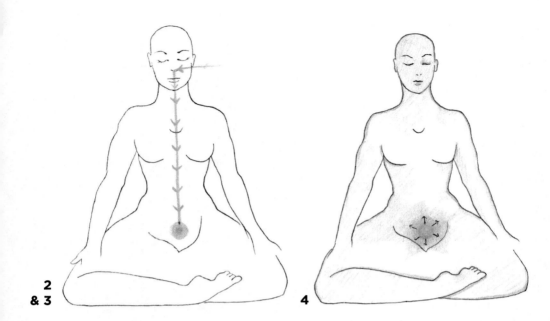

2 & 3

4

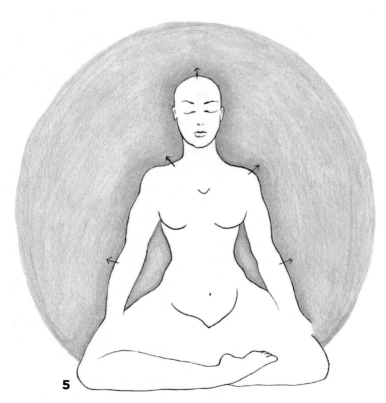

5

Note: Some people may feel dizzy when they start practicing Joshin Kokyu Hô. It's best to start with a few minutes and build this practice over time.

hands-on
healing
self-care protocol

The hands-on healing positions are an excellent structure to start establishing your practice. The more attention you pay to the hands position, the more meditative this practice becomes. Notice how, day by day, each position feels different. Notice how the various parts of your body feel when you place your hands on your head or belly. Notice when your entire body relaxes.

    In time, follow your instincts and personalize the hand positions to suit your needs. Remember, being in the space created by Reiki practice is more important than where your hands are placed.

how to prepare for self-care protocol

1.   Find a place where you will not be interrupted and sit comfortably (you may lie down, but that makes it's easier to fall asleep).

2.   Perform Kenyoku Hô to activate meridians and Joshin Kokyu Hô for a few breaths to center yourself.

3.   Recite the Reiki precepts. and set your intention of receiving what you need during yourReiki self-care session.

4.   Do the hands position with a meditative state of mind.

5.   Close with Gassho, to give thanks.

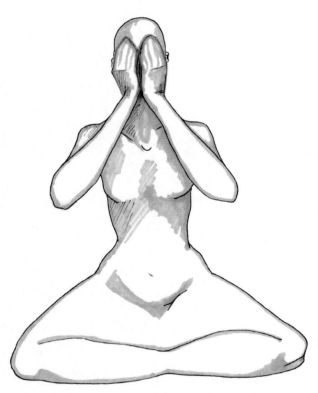

Position 1
eyes

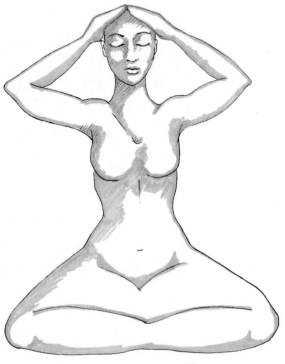

Position 2
top of the head

22

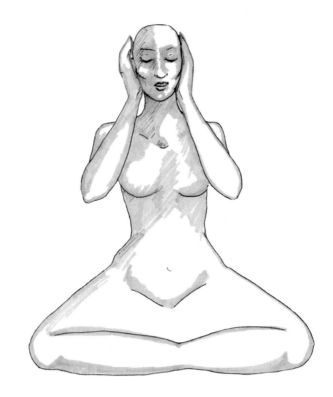

Position 3
ears

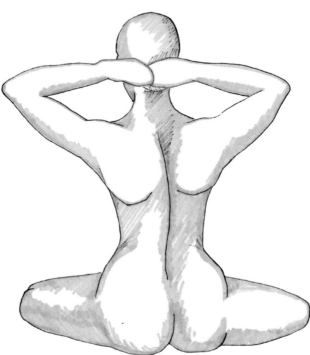

Position 4
back of the head

23

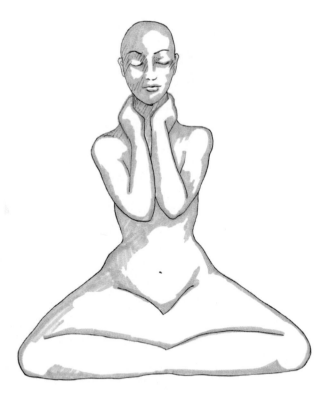

Position 5
throat

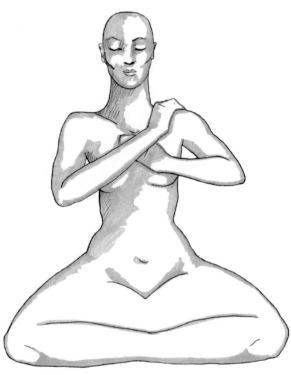

Position 6
left shoulder/
heart

24

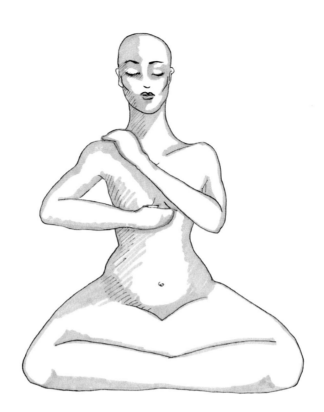

Position 7
right shoulder/
solar plexus

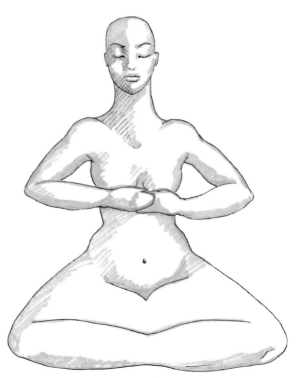

Position 8
front of the
body/core

25

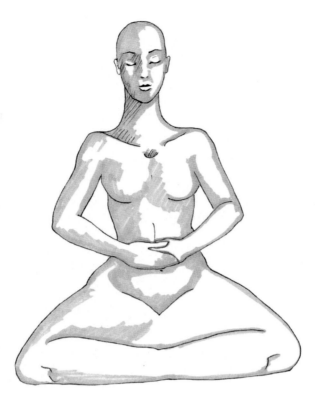

Position 9
abdomen

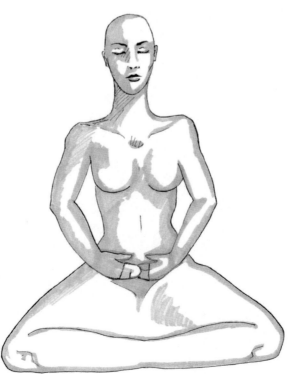

Position 10
lower abdomen

26

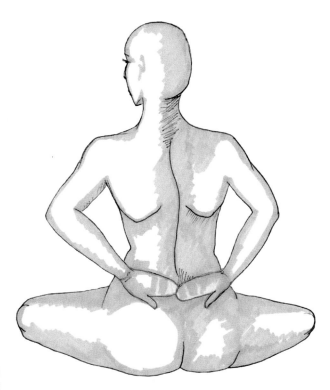

Position 11
lower back

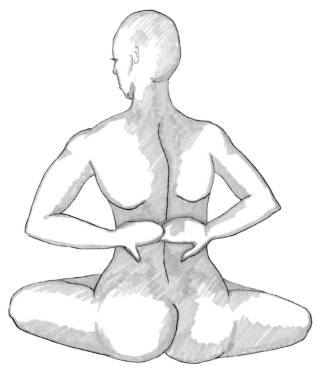

Position 12
mid-back

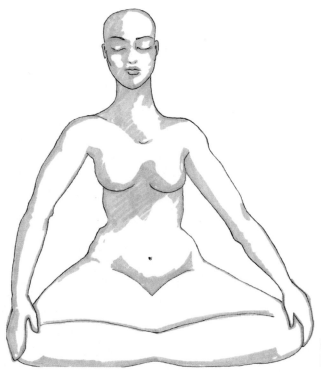

Position 13
knees

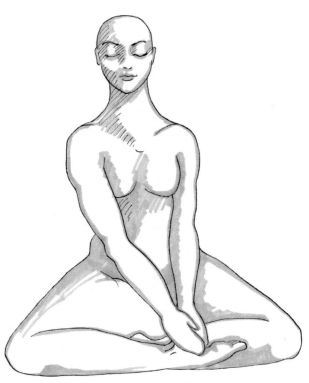

Position 14
feet

28

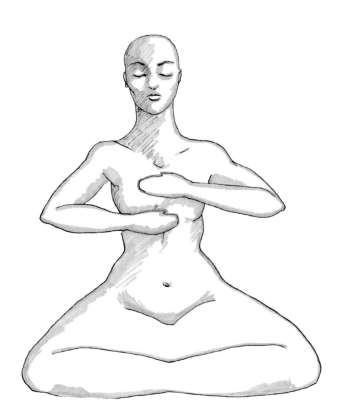

Position 15
universal
balancing
pose

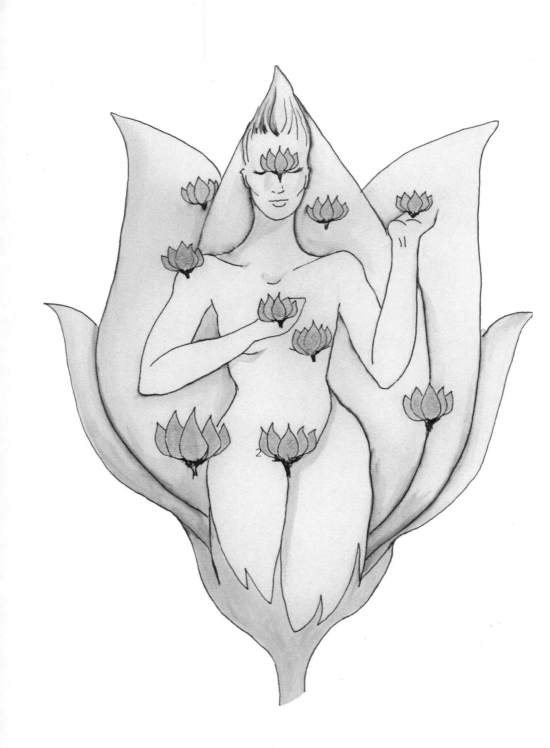

additional meditations

What defines Reiki practice? Is it only hands-on healing? Does it embody the precepts? The answer is personal. But if we went back to early-20th-century Japan, we'd find that spiritual practices included modalities such as meditation, visualizations and chanting. Mikao Usui was trained in esoteric Buddhism and other Japanese spiritual practices rich with tools that could help propel an individual's transformative journey forward beyond hands-on healing.

Besides Reiki, I practice Iaidō, the art of drawing the sword. And although mastering katas could be seen as the main objective of this particular martial art, the practice actually starts much earlier, and involves everything from how you greet others and put on your uniform to how you enter the dōjō and perform the Reijo (a ritual in which you become one with the sword/wisdom).

For me, Reiki practice informs everything I do in life: from how I react when the crap hits the fan, to performing hands-on healing, to that quiet moment in the evening when I like to explore Reiki-based meditations and visualizations. In the following chapters, you will find several meditations that are simple yet can, in my experience, bring about profound transformation. Use them to deepen your everyday practice.

seishin toitsu

The Japanese word "seishin" can be translated as "pure mind" or "spirit." "Toitsu" means gathering together, or focusing on the here and now.

When we practice the Seishin Toitsu meditation, we are aligning our breath and our mind, our spirit and our body, our heart and our Hara.

Seishin Toitsu is often practiced as one step of a more extended meditation called Hatsurei Hô (see page 41) but in itself is an effective concentration and meditation tool.

1.   Place your hands in Gassho and focus on the Hara. On the inhale, draw energy into your hands, feeling it moving up your arms and then down through your body and into the Hara.

2.   On the exhale, visualize energy moving from the Hara back up through the body, through the arms and then out through the hands.

3.   Repeat steps 1 to 2 as many times as you wish.

4.   Close with Gassho, to give thanks.

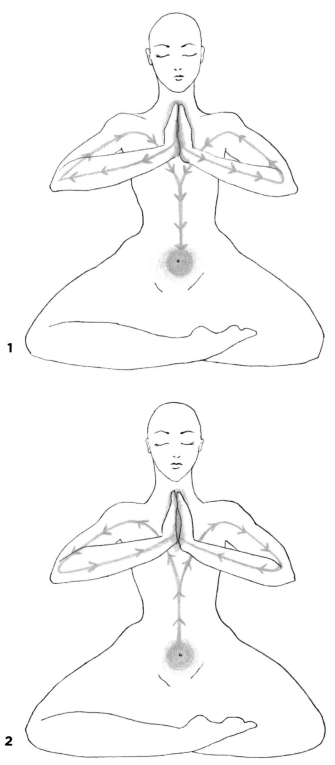

3 diamonds

Traditionally a Qigong technique, 3 diamonds may be combined with Reiki practice to connect the three energy centers.

1. Sit and place your hands in Gassho to center the mind and set the intent of connecting the 3 diamonds.

2. Place both hands approximately 4 inches from the body, over the Hara. Feel the connection.

3. Move both hands to the center of your chest (heart) and stay this way until you once again feel a connection. Imagine that you have connected the Hara with the heart center.

4. Move both hands to the forehead and stay this way until you once again feel a connection. Imagine that you have connected the heart with the mind.

5. Bring your hands to your heart center again and feel the connection.

6. Lower your hands to the Hara. You have now completed one cycle. Repeat steps 3 to 6 as many times as you wish.

7. Close with Gassho, to give thanks.

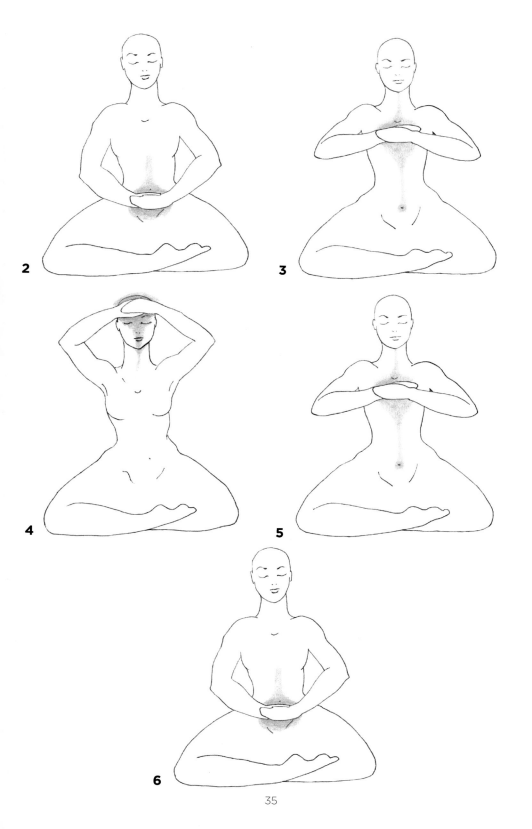

tanden chiryo-hô

This technique helps you balance your Heaven ki with your Earth ki, and to let go of negativity at the mental, physical, spiritual and emotional levels. It breaks down negative cycles and opens the door to new perspectives. It also promotes detoxification of the body (drink plenty of water afterward!).

1.   Sit comfortably and center yourself using Gassho.

2.   Set your intention to practice Tanden Chiryo-Hô and
        receive the benefits you need at the moment.

3.   Place one hand on the Hara and the other on your forehead.
        Notice any change in your hands, body or energy. Spend
        5 minutes in this position.

4.   Lower the hand that is on your forehead and place it over
        the hand that is on the Hara. Notice any change in your
        hands, body or energy. Stay in this position for approxi-
        mately 15 minutes. Feel the grounding effect and the
        support of your hands on the Hara.

5.   Close with Gassho, to give thanks.

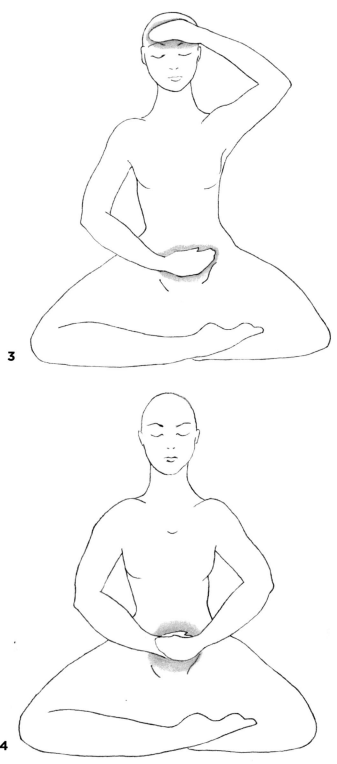

3

4

reiki shower

Reiki showers are often introduced as a modality to cleanse negative energy picked up from others from the astral body, but this concept doesn't fit in the framework of traditional Japanese Reiki practice—if we follow the precept of "Do not worry," there is no need for protection. If we have a strong Hara and are grounded in ourselves, we don't feel the need to protect our energy from others and aren't afraid of picking up negative vibes (if we feel like we need to protect, we are worrying). However, Reiki showers are a way of centering ourselves in our body, as well as a way of cultivating our awareness of energy.

1. Stand or sit comfortably, your back straight. Place your hands in Gassho and set the intention to receive whatever you need to receive.

2. Raise your arms vertically, hands above your head, palms facing each other. Visualize a white light between your hands.

3. Move your hands slowly down the front of the body, palms facing the body. Visualize the white light coming from your palms, showering your body. Feel the energy. Swipe your hands over your thighs and visualize the light going into the earth.

4. Repeat steps 2 to 5 twice.

5. Close with Gassho, to give thanks.

This how-to doesn't include the symbols (see page 46), but if you wish to add them, you can do so in one of two ways: (1) During step 2, visualize each symbol and repeat its mantra three times, then move on to step 3. (2) Work with one symbol at the time; that is, visualize the first symbol and say its mantra three times on step 2, move on to step 3, then repeat with the other three symbols, for a total of four passes.

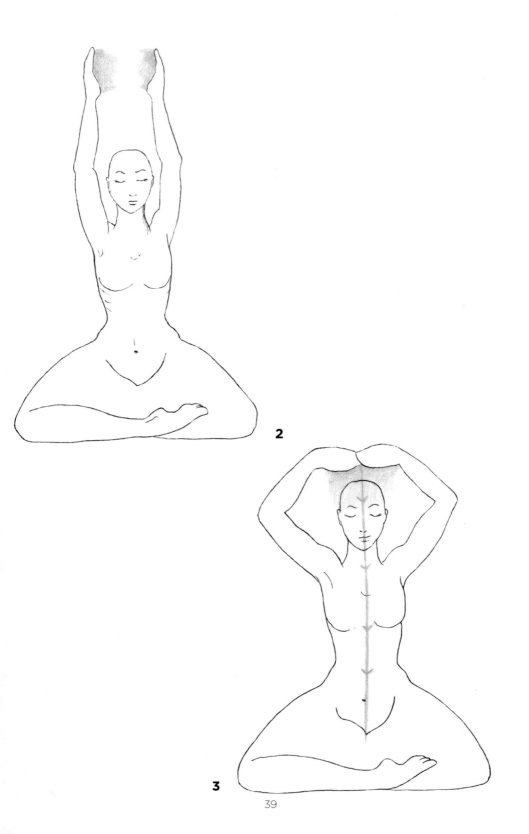

2

3

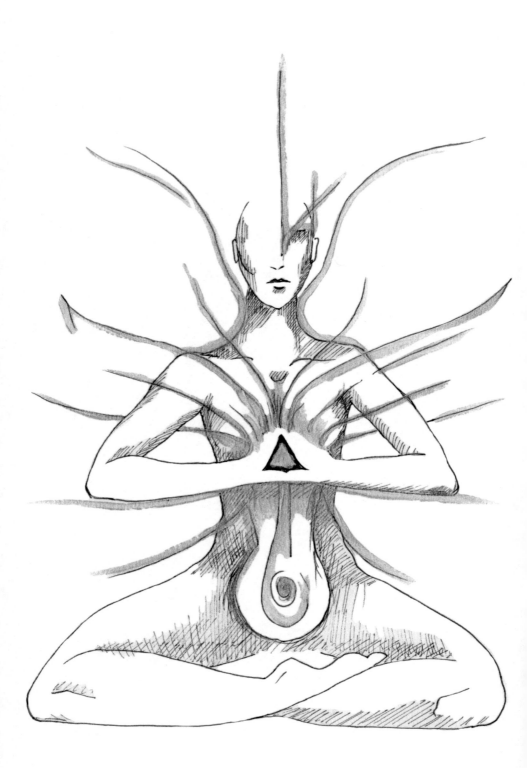

hatsurei hô

Traditionally taught during Okuden (Reiki Level II), Hatsurei Hô includes several meditations and techniques that are shown earlier in the book, such as Gassho, Kenyoku Hô, Joshin Kokyu Hô and Seishin Toitsu, and, when practiced in Japan, the precepts.

In Japanese, "Hatsu" means to bring forth, to reveal. "Rei" means spirit and spiritual ability, and "Hô" can be translated as "method." So we can see this meditation as "the method to bring forth your hidden spiritual ability"—but also as a beautiful amalgamation of the essential teachings of Reiki practice, meditating on the precepts, grounding ourselves in our body, strengthening our Hara and connecting it to our Heart and Heaven ki centers.

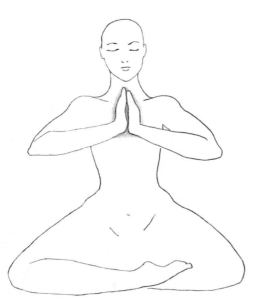

1. Place your hands in Gassho to set your intention to perform Hatsurei Hô. Recite or meditate with the Precepts.

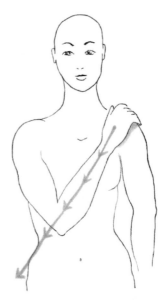

2a. Kenyoku Hô: Place your right hand on your left shoulder. Inhale. On the exhale, sweep downward diagonally from the left shoulder to the right hip.

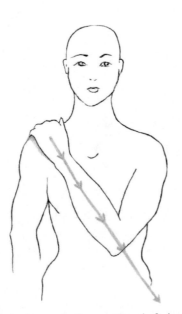

2b. Inhale and place your left hand on the right shoulder. Exhale and sweep downward diagonally from the right shoulder to the left hip.

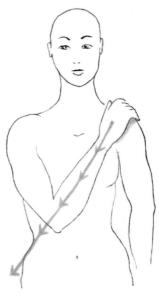

2c. Inhale as you return your right hand to your left shoulder. On the exhale, sweep diagonally down from the left shoulder to the right hip.

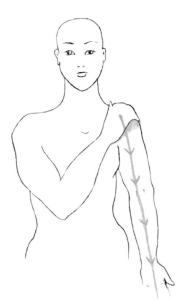

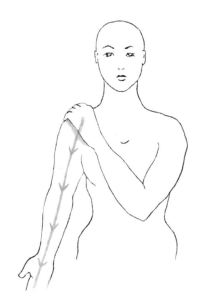

2d. With the left elbow against your side and your arm perpendicular to the ground, place your right hand on the left shoulder. Inhale and exhale as you sweep downward to the left fingertips.

2e. With the right elbow against your side and arm perpendicular to the ground, place your left hand on the right shoulder. Inhale and exhale as you sweep downward to the right fingertips.

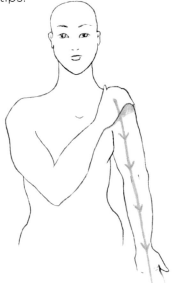

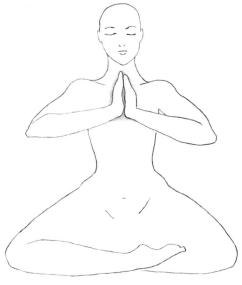

2f. With the left elbow against your side and your arm perpendicular to the ground, place your right hand on the left shoulder. Inhale and exhale as you sweep downward to the left fingertips.

3. Place your hands in Gassho and set your intent to perform Joshin Kokyu Hô.

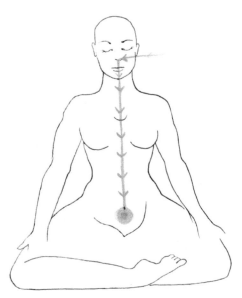

4a. Joshin Kokyu Hô: Close your eyes and place your hands on your thighs, palms facing upward. Inhale, feeling the energy coming in through the nose and moving down to the Hara.

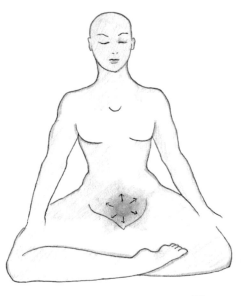

4b. Pause, feeling the energy fill your entire body.

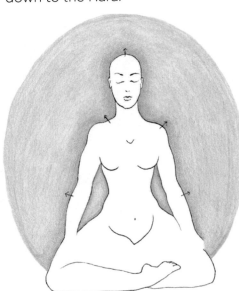

4c. Exhale, expanding the energy out of the body through every pore, into your surroundings. Repeat this cycle for a few minutes.

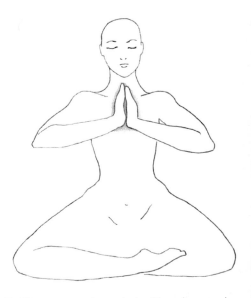

5. Place your hands in Gassho and set your intent to perform Seishin Toitsu.

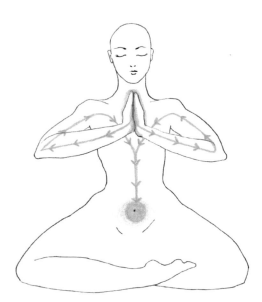

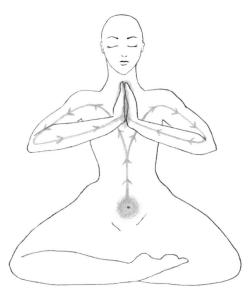

6a. Seishin Toitsu: On the inhale, draw energy into your hands, feeling it moving along your arms, down though your body and into the Hara.

6b. On the exhale, visualize energy moving from the Hara back up through the body, through the arms and then out through the hands. Repeat this cycle for a few minutes.

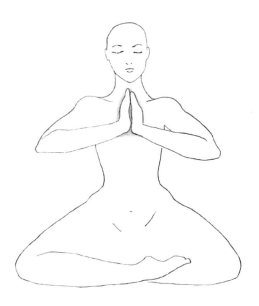

7. Close with Gassho, to give thanks.

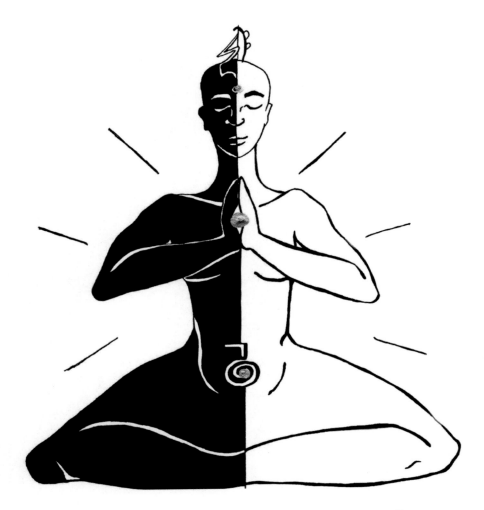

working with the symbols and mantras

Traditional Japanese Reiki practice has four symbols and mantras: three learned during Okuden (Reiki Level II), and one during Shinpiden (Reiki Level III). Although people refer to the symbols by their mantras, they are different tools.

symbol 1

Mantra: Choku Rei

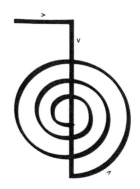

The words "Choku Rei" can be interpreted as going back to your true self, as "being direct" or as "straight spirit." The mantra and its symbol are associated with Earth ki: focused, powerful and grounding. When we are grounded, we are less afraid, less worried and more honest with ourselves and others. Working with Choku Rei stimulates the Hara and your connection to life.

symbol 2

Mantra: Sei Heki

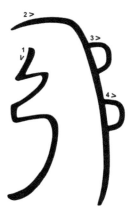

The mantra "Sei Heki" can be translated as "mental habit," or the habitual inclination to rediscover the inner essence of one's true nature. It's associated with harmony and heavenly energy, which is lighter than Earth ki. Practicing with this mantra or symbol helps boost our intuition and our spiritual connection. It can also increase our psychic ability.

symbol 3

Mantra: Hon Sha Ze Sho Nen

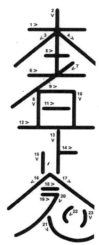

The symbol is, in reality, the compression of five kanjis, which can be translated as "My original nature is correct thought" or "I am right mindfulness." It's associated with heart energy, and it reminds us of our interconnectedness (oneness) with everything. It's used for remote sessions, because when we remember we are all one, we create a space where distance doesn't exist.

symbol 4

Mantra: Dai Kômyô

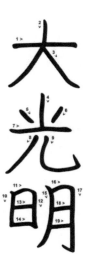

The symbol consists of three kanjis, which can be translated as "big, bright light." It represents the pure light of our true essence (Buddha nature) and the state of mind of enlightenment.

The bottom two kanjis represent the sun and the moon respectively, and stand for absolute truth. Their coming together also symbolizes non-duality.

meditating with the symbols

I was taught in Reiki II to use the Reiki symbols during my sessions. Although drawing them in the air or on my palms got me into the "right space" for a treatment, I never felt comfortable with this style. I'm more of a minimalist, and feel shy when it comes to movement (but once you get me talking, beware!). I think that's why the simplicity of the Japanese approach is so attractive to me. Yes, it requires more discipline: I have to meditate on the symbols and integrate their energies, but I can let go during sessions and just hold the space for my clients so they can take whatever they need.

The beauty of Reiki practice having many tools and approaches is that we can all find a tool or style that suits our personality. In this section, I share modalities to work with the symbols beyond the sessions. There are many more, but these ones are simple, and easy to integrate into your daily practice.

stepping into the symbols

1. Standing, draw a symbol with your palm (palm facing outward). Keep the other hand on the Hara.

2. Repeat the symbol's mantra three times.

3. Step into the space of the symbol (arms down along your sides) and feel its energy.

Note: You may repeat this as many times as you wish, to work with one kind of energy. Or do each symbol in succession, to notice the subtle differences between their energies.

visualizing the symbols

1.   Sit comfortably, with your back straight.

2   Close your eyes, and visualize the symbol either in front of you or inside your entire body.

3.   Repeat its mantra three times.

4.   Feel and observe its energy, without judgment.

Note: You may repeat this as many times as you wish, to work with one kind of energy. Or do each symbol in succession, to notice the subtle differences between their energies.

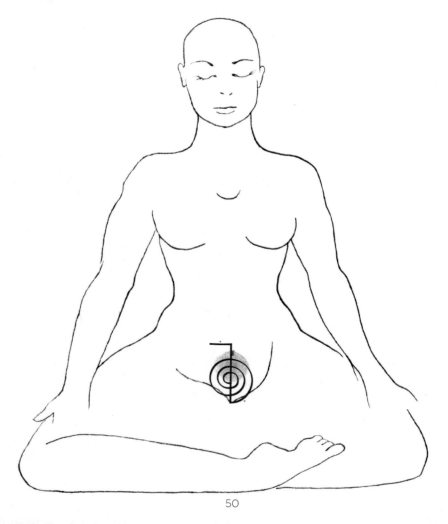

visualizing the symbols in the hara

1. Sit with your back straight, hands on your thighs, palms facing upward.

2. Choose a symbol to work with.

3. Visualize a bright sphere of light in the Hara, with the symbol inside it.

4. Breathe normally and keep your awareness on the bright sphere of light containing the symbol.

5. Do this for a few minutes and then notice the space you created.

chanting the mantras

1. Sit or stand with your feet planted firmly on the ground.

2. Choose a mantra to work with. You can use the entire mantra or just the vowels (see chart below).

3. Inhale all the way to the Hara, then exhale, chanting the mantra from the Hara. Feel how your entire body vibrates with the sound.

4. Chant for as long as you wish, and then remain in the space you created. Notice how it affects you.

Choku Rei:	o-u-e-i
Sei Heki:	e-i-e-ki
Hon Sha Ze Sho Nen:	o-a-ze-o-ney
Dai Kômyô:	a-i-ko-yo

bright spheres

"Dai Kômyô," the mantra associated with the fourth symbol, can be translated as "big, bright light"—the one that represents our true, non-dual nature. I learned this meditation from Frans Stiene, and to this day it's still one of my favorites. If you have not learned the fourth symbol, you can do this meditation using just the bright spheres of light.

1. Sit comfortably, with your back straight, hands on your thighs, palms facing upward.

2. Place your hands in Gassho to set your intention to receive whatever you need during this meditation.

3. Close your eyes and visualize a bright sphere of light over your head.

4. Visualize another bright sphere over your right shoulder.

5. Visualize another bright sphere over your left shoulder.

6. Visualize another bright sphere in your head, at the height of your forehead.

7. Visualize another bright sphere in your head, behind your nose/mouth area.

8. Visualize another bright sphere over your right hand.

9. Visualize another bright sphere over your left hand.

10. Visualize another bright sphere inside your heart area.
    This bright sphere contains the fourth symbol (Dai Kômyô).

11. Inhale and feel all the bright spheres moving toward the
    one in the heart area, and becoming one big, bright sphere
    of light, with the fourth symbol in its middle.

12. Inhale and let that big, bright sphere of light become one with
    your body.

13. Stay in the space you created for a few moments.

14. Close with Gassho, to give thanks.

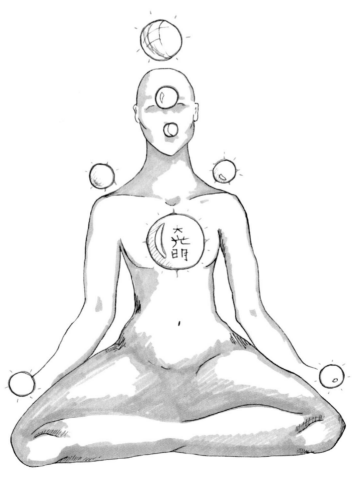

heartfelt
thank-yous

Thank you to my teachers, and especially to Frans Stiene for showing me the way to a deeper practice and for taking the time to read my manuscript, make sure I didn't include anything slightly insane and write a beautiful foreword.

Thank you, Silvia Colsher, for being there always, and the beautiful art direction. To Judy Phillips, for making sure my English is truly English and not SpanFrenGlish. And to Aura Sosa for making me look great in my author photo.

Thank you to The Pack, my family, my dōjō tribe and all my awesome friends and mermaids for listening to my rambling, and for acting as willing guinea pigs. I heart you all from here to the moon. And thank you to my Reiki colleagues, students and clients, who have been the wonderful teachers in this beautiful journey.

about nathalie

Nathalie Jaspar is a writer, illustrator and Reiki master based in New York City. She's certified by the International House of Reiki, led by world-renowned Reiki master Frans Stiene. She also trained at the Center for True Health, at the International Center for Reiki and with Reiki master Pamela Miles at the JCC Reiki Clinic in New York City.

Nathalie is passionate about sharing new ways to experience Reiki practice beyond hands-on healing, including through meditations, breathing modalities and visualizations, which work wonders in everyday life. As well as offering sessions and workshops in New York, Nathalie has been invited to demonstrate Reiki practice in venues as diverse as advertising agencies, Fashion Week events and the New York Jets' Atlantic Health Training Center.

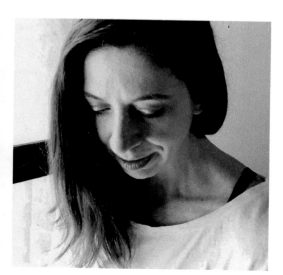

Nathalie's lineage
Usui Mikao
Kanichi Taketomi
Kimiko Koyama
Doi Hiroshi
Frans Stiene
Deborah Flanagan
Nathalie Jaspar

Made in the USA
Las Vegas, NV
03 July 2022

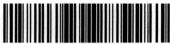

51043174R00040